IVF DIET COOKBOOK

Dr. Kimberly Carlos

Copyright © 2023 by Dr. Kimberly Carlos

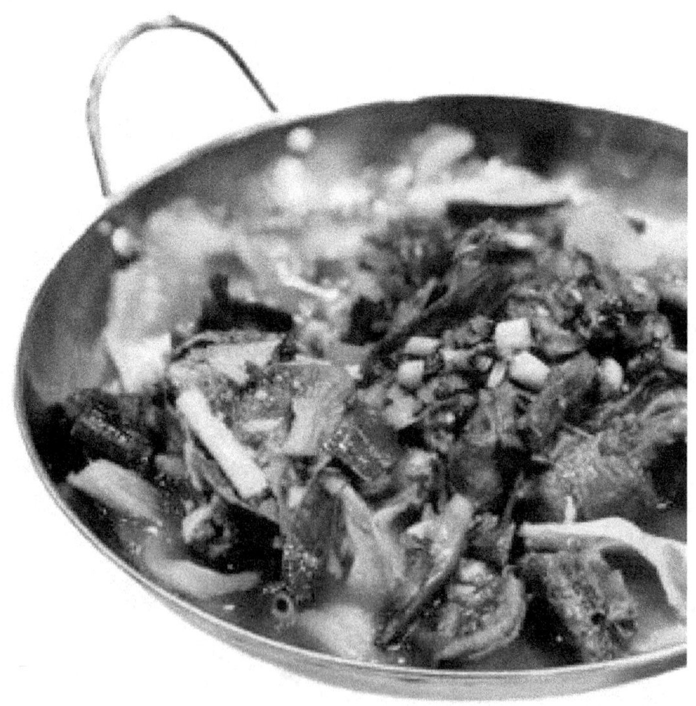

TABLE OF CONTENT

CHAPTER ONE

Following an IVF (In Vitro Fertilization) diet with Benefits

Following an IVF (In Vitro Fertilization) diet can be beneficial for individuals undergoing fertility treatments, as it may help optimize their chances of a successful pregnancy. Keep in mind that you should consult with a healthcare professional or a registered dietitian before making any significant dietary changes, as individual needs and recommendations can vary.

Here's a general guideline for following an IVF diet with potential benefits:

1. Eat a Balanced Diet:

- Focus on a well-balanced diet that includes a variety of nutrient-rich foods from all food groups.
- Aim for a mix of fruits, vegetables, whole grains, lean proteins, and healthy fats.

2. Increase Folate Intake:

- Folate is essential for fetal development, so consider

adding folate-rich foods to your diet.

- Sources of folate include leafy greens, citrus fruits, fortified cereals, and legumes.

3. Omega-3 Fatty Acids: Omega-3 fatty acids, found in fatty fish (like salmon and mackerel), flaxseeds, and walnuts, may help support fertility and reduce inflammation.

4. Antioxidant-Rich Foods: Antioxidants can protect eggs and sperm from oxidative stress. Include foods like berries, nuts, seeds, and colorful vegetables in your diet.

5. Limit Processed Foods and Sugar: Avoid or limit processed foods, sugary snacks, and drinks, as they can lead to weight gain and insulin resistance, which may affect fertility.

6. Maintain a Healthy Weight: Achieving and maintaining a healthy weight is important for fertility. Both obesity and being underweight can impact fertility.

7. Protein Sources:

- Choose lean protein sources like poultry, fish, beans, and tofu over red meat.
- Plant-based proteins can be a good choice, but make

sure you get a variety of amino acids through a mix of plant sources.

8. Limit Caffeine and Alcohol: High caffeine and alcohol consumption may negatively impact fertility. Limit both to moderate levels or as recommended by your healthcare provider.

9. Stay Hydrated: Proper hydration is essential for overall health. Drink plenty of water throughout the day.

10. Whole Grains: Opt for whole grains like quinoa, brown rice, and whole wheat pasta over refined grains to help regulate blood sugar levels.

11. Calcium and Vitamin D: Ensure adequate intake of calcium and vitamin D for bone health. Dairy products, fortified non-dairy alternatives, and leafy greens are good sources.

12. Supplements: Talk to your healthcare provider about any supplements, such as folic acid, prenatal vitamins, or specific fertility supplements, that may be recommended for you.

13. Manage Stress: Stress can negatively affect fertility, so consider stress-reduction techniques like meditation, yoga, or counseling.

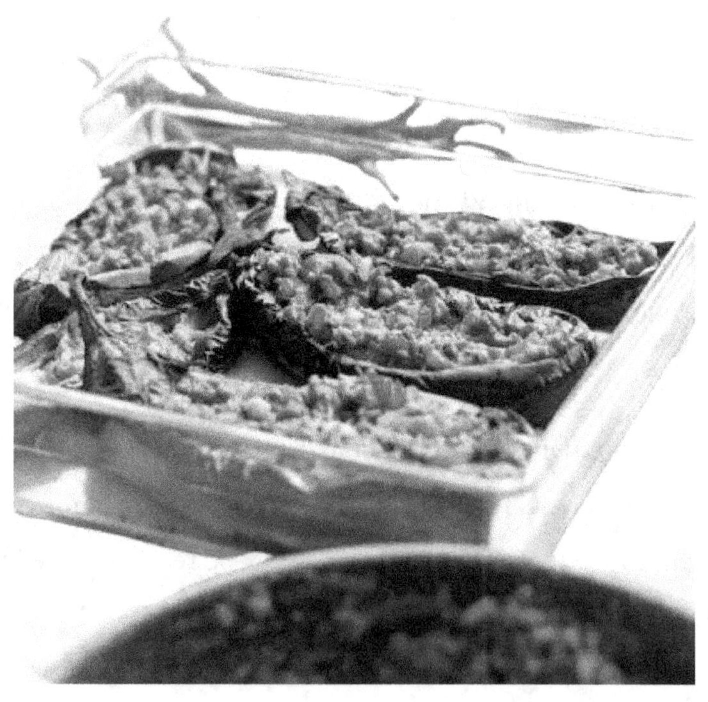

CHAPTER TWO

A 14-Day IVF Diet Meal Plan

Day 1

- **Breakfast:** Greek yogurt with berries and a sprinkle of flaxseeds.
- **Lunch:** Grilled chicken breast with quinoa and steamed broccoli.
- **Snack:** Carrot sticks with hummus.
- **Dinner:** Baked salmon with asparagus and a side salad.

Day 2

- **Breakfast:** Spinach and mushroom omelet with whole-grain toast.
- **Lunch:** Lentil and vegetable soup with a side of mixed greens.
- **Snack:** Almonds and a small apple.
- Dinner: Turkey chili with brown rice.

Day 3

- **Breakfast:** Oatmeal topped with sliced bananas and chopped walnuts.

- **Lunch:** Tuna salad with mixed greens and whole-grain crackers.
- **Snack:** Greek yogurt and a handful of mixed berries.
- **Dinner:** Grilled shrimp with quinoa and roasted Brussels sprouts.

Day 4

- Breakfast: Smoothie with spinach, frozen berries, almond milk, and a scoop of protein powder.
- Lunch: Chickpea and vegetable stir-fry with brown rice.
- Snack: Cottage cheese with pineapple chunks.
- Dinner: Baked chicken thighs with sweet potato and green beans.

Day 5

- **Breakfast:** Whole-grain waffles with fresh strawberries and a dollop of Greek yogurt.
- **Lunch:** Spinach and feta stuffed bell peppers.
- **Snack:** Sliced cucumber with tzatziki sauce.
- **Dinner:** Grilled tofu with quinoa and roasted asparagus.

Day 6

- **Breakfast:** Scrambled eggs with sautéed spinach and whole-grain toast.
- **Lunch:** Turkey and avocado wrap with a side of carrot sticks.
- **Snack:** Mixed nuts and dried apricots.
- **Dinner:** Baked cod with brown rice and steamed broccoli.

Day 7:

- **Breakfast:** Cottage cheese parfait with sliced peaches and honey.
- **Lunch:** Quinoa salad with chickpeas, cherry tomatoes, and cucumber.
- **Snack:** Sliced bell peppers with guacamole.
- **Dinner:** Beef and vegetable kebabs with a quinoa pilaf.

Day 8

- **Breakfast:** Smoothie with kale, banana, chia seeds, and almond milk.
- **Lunch:** Quinoa and black bean salad with a lime-cilantro dressing.

- **Snack:** Sliced mango with a sprinkle of Tajin seasoning.
- **Dinner:** Grilled chicken with a side of roasted butternut squash and sautéed spinach.

Day 9

- **Breakfast:** Whole-grain pancakes with blueberries and a dollop of low-fat ricotta cheese.
- **Lunch:** Lentil and vegetable curry with brown rice.
- **Snack:** Celery sticks with almond butter.
- **Dinner:** Baked cod with a quinoa and mixed vegetable medley.

Day 10

- Breakfast: Scrambled eggs with diced bell peppers and a slice of whole-grain toast.
- Lunch: Turkey and vegetable stir-fry with quinoa.
- Snack: A small handful of grapes and a string cheese.
- Dinner: Grilled shrimp with a side of roasted Brussels sprouts and sweet potato.

Day 11

- **Breakfast:** Greek yogurt parfait with granola and mixed berries.
- **Lunch:** Spinach and artichoke stuffed chicken breast with a side of asparagus.
- **Snack:** Sliced pear with a drizzle of honey.
- **Dinner:** Baked tofu with a quinoa and broccoli salad.

Day 12

- **Breakfast:** Spinach and tomato frittata with a whole-grain English muffin.
- **Lunch:** Chickpea and cucumber salad with a lemon-tahini dressing.
- **Snack:** Trail mix with almonds, dried cranberries, and pumpkin seeds.
- **Dinner:** Beef or plant-based patty with a lettuce wrap and roasted sweet potato fries.

Day 13

- **Breakfast:** Oatmeal with diced apples, cinnamon, and a dollop of almond butter.
- **Lunch:** Turkey and avocado salad with mixed greens and balsamic vinaigrette.

- **Snack:** Cottage cheese with sliced kiwi.
- **Dinner:** Baked salmon with quinoa and roasted broccoli.

Day 14

- **Breakfast:** Smoothie with spinach, frozen mixed berries, chia seeds, and coconut water.
- **Lunch:** Quinoa and vegetable bowl with a tahini dressing.
- **Snack:** Sliced bell peppers with guacamole.
- **Dinner:** Grilled chicken or tofu with a side of brown rice and sautéed kale.

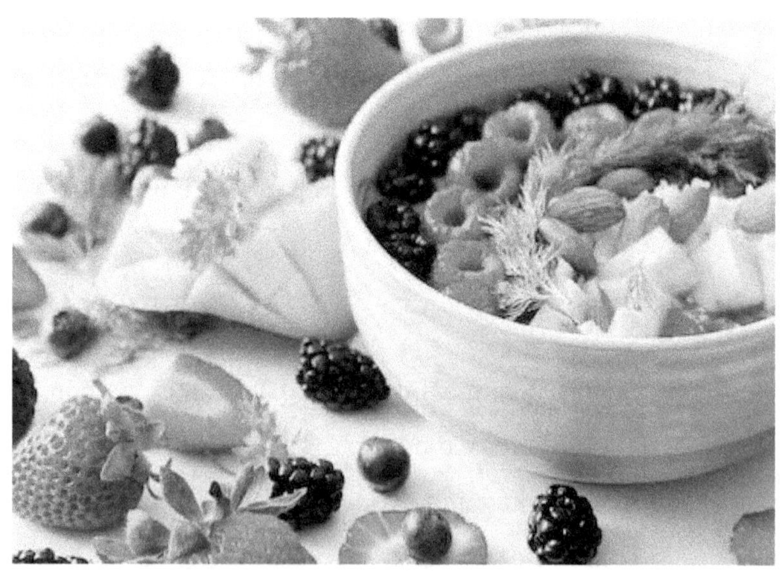

CHAPTER THREE

IVF Diet Breakfast Recipes

1. Greek Yogurt Parfait

This Greek yogurt parfait is rich in protein and probiotics, making it a great choice for a healthy IVF diet breakfast.

Ingredients:

- 1 cup Greek yogurt
- 1/2 cup fresh mixed berries
- 2 tablespoons honey or maple syrup
- 1/4 cup granola

Instructions:

1. In a bowl or glass, layer Greek yogurt, berries, and honey or maple syrup.

2. Top with granola for added crunch.

3. Serve immediately.

Cooking Time: 5 minutes

2. Spinach and Mushroom Omelet

Packed with folate and protein, this spinach and mushroom omelet is a nutritious choice for an IVF diet breakfast.

Ingredients:

- 2 large eggs
- 1/4 cup chopped spinach
- 1/4 cup sliced mushrooms
- Salt and pepper to taste
- 1 teaspoon olive oil

Instructions:

1. In a bowl, whisk the eggs and season with salt and pepper.

2. Heat olive oil in a non-stick skillet over medium heat.

3. Add mushrooms and sauté until tender, then add spinach.

4. Pour the whisked eggs over the veggies and cook until set, then fold in half.

5. Serve hot.

Cooking Time: 10 minutes

3. Berry and Spinach Smoothie

This green smoothie is packed with vitamins, antioxidants, and fertility-boosting ingredients.

Ingredients:

- 1 cup spinach leaves
- 1/2 cup mixed berries (fresh or frozen)
- 1 banana
- 1 cup almond milk (or any milk of your choice)
- 1 tablespoon chia seeds

Instructions:

1. Place all ingredients in a blender.

2. Blend until smooth and creamy.

3. Pour into a glass and enjoy immediately.

Cooking Time: 5 minutes

4. Quinoa Breakfast Bowl

A protein-rich quinoa breakfast bowl with nuts and fruits is a filling and nutritious choice for IVF diet breakfast.

Ingredients:

- 1/2 cup cooked quinoa
- 1/4 cup chopped almonds or walnuts
- 1/4 cup mixed fresh fruits (e.g., apples, berries, bananas)
- 1 tablespoon honey or maple syrup
- 1/4 teaspoon cinnamon (optional)

Instructions:

1. In a bowl, combine quinoa, nuts, and fruits.

2. Drizzle with honey or maple syrup and sprinkle with cinnamon if desired.

3. Mix well and serve.

Cooking Time: 10 minutes (for cooking quinoa)

5. Overnight Oats

Prepare this IVF diet-friendly breakfast the night before for a quick and easy morning meal.

Ingredients:

- 1/2 cup rolled oats

- 1/2 cup Greek yogurt
- 1/2 cup almond milk (or any milk of your choice)
- 1 tablespoon chia seeds
- 1/2 cup mixed berries
- 1 tablespoon honey or maple syrup

Instructions:

1. In a jar or container, combine oats, yogurt, milk, and chia seeds.

2. Add berries and sweeten with honey or maple syrup.

3. Stir well, cover, and refrigerate overnight.

4. Enjoy in the morning.

Cooking Time: None (requires overnight refrigeration)

6. Avocado and Tomato Toast

Avocado and tomato toast is a simple yet nutritious breakfast option, rich in healthy fats and vitamins.

Ingredients:

- 2 slices of whole-grain bread
- 1 ripe avocado

- 1 medium tomato, sliced

- Salt and pepper to taste

- Optional toppings: red pepper flakes, sliced radishes

Instructions:

1. Toast the bread until it's crispy.

2. Mash the avocado and spread it evenly on the toasted bread.

3. Top with tomato slices and season with salt and pepper.

4. Add optional toppings if desired.

5. Serve immediately.

Cooking Time: 5 minutes

7. Peanut Butter and Banana Smoothie

This smoothie combines the richness of peanut butter with the natural sweetness of bananas for a delicious and filling IVF diet breakfast.

Ingredients:

- 1 ripe banana

- 2 tablespoons natural peanut butter

- 1 cup almond milk (or any milk of your choice)

- 1 tablespoon honey or maple syrup

- Ice cubes (optional)

Instructions:

1. Place all ingredients in a blender.

2. Blend until smooth and creamy.

3. Add ice cubes if you prefer a colder smoothie.

4. Pour into a glass and enjoy.

Cooking Time: 5 minutes

8. Chia Seed Pudding

Chia seed pudding is a versatile and nutrient-packed breakfast that can be customized with your favorite toppings.

Ingredients:

- 2 tablespoons chia seeds

- 1 cup almond milk (or any milk of your choice)

- 1 tablespoon honey or maple syrup

- Fresh berries or sliced fruit for topping

Instructions:

1. In a jar or container, combine chia seeds, almond milk, and honey or maple syrup.

2. Stir well, cover, and refrigerate for at least 2 hours or overnight.

3. Before serving, top with fresh berries or fruit.

Cooking Time: 2 hours (for pudding to set)

9. Sweet Potato and Spinach Breakfast Hash

This savory breakfast hash is loaded with nutrients from sweet potatoes and spinach.

Ingredients:

- 1 medium sweet potato, diced
- 1 cup fresh spinach leaves
- 2 eggs
- Salt and pepper to taste
- 1 tablespoon olive oil

Instructions:

1. Heat olive oil in a skillet over medium heat.

2. Add diced sweet potatoes and cook until they become tender and slightly crispy.

3. Stir in fresh spinach and cook until wilted.

4. Make two wells in the mixture and crack eggs into them.

5. Cook until the egg whites are set but the yolks are still runny.

6. Season with salt and pepper and serve hot.

Cooking Time: 20 minutes

10. Cottage Cheese and Fruit Bowl

A cottage cheese and fruit bowl is a quick, protein-rich breakfast option.

Ingredients:

- 1/2 cup low-fat cottage cheese
- 1/2 cup mixed fresh fruit (e.g., pineapple, strawberries, kiwi)
- 1 tablespoon honey or maple syrup
- 1/4 cup chopped nuts (e.g., almonds, walnuts)

Instructions:

1. In a bowl, combine cottage cheese and fresh fruit.

2. Drizzle with honey or maple syrup and sprinkle with chopped nuts.

3. Mix well and serve.

Cooking Time: 5 minutes.

IVF Diet Lunch Recipes

1. Quinoa and Chickpea Salad

This quinoa and chickpea salad is a nutrient-packed lunch option that provides protein, fiber, and essential vitamins and minerals.

Ingredients:

- 1 cup cooked quinoa
- 1 cup canned chickpeas, drained and rinsed
- 1 cup diced cucumber
- 1 cup diced bell peppers
- 1/4 cup chopped fresh parsley
- Juice of 1 lemon
- 2 tablespoons olive oil
- Salt and pepper to taste

Instructions:

1. In a large bowl, combine quinoa, chickpeas, cucumber, bell peppers, and fresh parsley.

2. In a separate small bowl, whisk together lemon juice, olive oil, salt, and pepper.

3. Pour the dressing over the salad and toss to combine.

4. Serve chilled.

Cooking Time: 15 minutes (for cooking quinoa)

2. Spinach and Feta Stuffed Bell Peppers

These stuffed bell peppers are packed with folate, iron, and protein, making them an ideal IVF diet lunch option.

Ingredients:

- 2 large bell peppers (any color)
- 1 cup cooked quinoa
- 1 cup fresh spinach, chopped
- 1/2 cup crumbled feta cheese
- 1/4 cup diced tomatoes
- 1/4 cup diced red onion

-   1 teaspoon olive oil

-   Salt and pepper to taste

Instructions:

1. Preheat the oven to 375°F (190°C).

2. Cut the tops off the bell peppers and remove seeds and membranes.

3. In a skillet, heat olive oil over medium heat and sauté the spinach until wilted.

4. In a bowl, combine quinoa, sautéed spinach, feta cheese, diced tomatoes, diced red onion, salt, and pepper.

5. Stuff the bell peppers with the quinoa mixture.

6. Place the stuffed peppers in a baking dish, cover with foil, and bake for about 25-30 minutes, or until the peppers are tender.

7. Serve hot.

Cooking Time: 30 minutes

3. Lentil and Vegetable Soup

This hearty lentil and vegetable soup is rich in fiber and plant-based protein, providing essential nutrients for your IVF diet.

Ingredients:

- 1 cup dried green or brown lentils, rinsed and drained
- 4 cups vegetable broth
- 1 cup diced carrots
- 1 cup diced celery
- 1 cup diced onion
- 2 cloves garlic, minced
- 1 teaspoon olive oil
- 1 bay leaf
- Salt and pepper to taste

Instructions:

1. In a large pot, heat olive oil over medium heat.

2. Add diced onion, carrots, and celery and sauté until softened.

3. Add minced garlic and cook for another minute.

4. Add lentils, vegetable broth, bay leaf, salt, and pepper.

5. Bring to a boil, then reduce heat, cover, and simmer for about 25-30 minutes, or until lentils are tender.

6. Remove the bay leaf before serving.

Cooking Time: 40 minutes

4. Tuna Salad Lettuce Wraps

Tuna salad lettuce wraps offer a protein-rich and low-carb lunch option suitable for your IVF diet.

Ingredients:

- 1 can (5 oz) tuna in water, drained
- 2 tablespoons Greek yogurt
- 1 tablespoon Dijon mustard
- 1/4 cup diced celery
- 1/4 cup diced red onion
- 1 tablespoon chopped fresh dill (or 1/2 teaspoon dried dill)
- Salt and pepper to taste
- Large lettuce leaves (e.g., iceberg or romaine)

Instructions:

1. In a bowl, combine drained tuna, Greek yogurt, Dijon mustard, diced celery, diced red onion, chopped dill, salt, and pepper.

2. Mix well until all ingredients are incorporated.

3. Spoon the tuna salad onto large lettuce leaves.

4. Roll up the lettuce leaves to form wraps.

5. Serve immediately.

Cooking Time: None

5. Turkey and Avocado Wrap

This turkey and avocado wrap is a protein-packed and satisfying lunch option for your IVF diet.

Ingredients:

- 2 whole-grain or spinach tortillas
- 4 slices turkey breast
- 1/2 avocado, sliced
- 1/2 cup mixed greens
- 2 tablespoons Greek yogurt or hummus (as a spread)
- Optional additions: sliced cucumber, bell peppers

Instructions:

1. Lay out the tortillas and spread Greek yogurt or hummus over them.

2. Layer turkey slices, avocado, mixed greens, and any

optional additions on each tortilla.

3. Roll up the tortillas tightly.

4. Cut each wrap in half diagonally.

5. Serve immediately.

Cooking Time: None

6. Chickpea and Vegetable Stir-Fry

A chickpea and vegetable stir-fry is a flavorful and protein-rich lunch option for your IVF diet.

Ingredients:

- 1 can (15 oz) chickpeas, drained and rinsed
- 2 cups mixed vegetables (e.g., bell peppers, broccoli, snap peas)
- 2 cloves garlic, minced
- 2 tablespoons low-sodium soy sauce or tamari
- 1 tablespoon olive oil
- 1 teaspoon grated ginger
- Optional toppings: sesame seeds, chopped green onions

Instructions:

1. Heat olive oil in a large skillet or wok over medium-high heat.

2. Add minced garlic and grated ginger and stir-fry for about 30 seconds.

3. Add mixed vegetables and cook until they become tender-crisp.

4. Stir in chickpeas and soy sauce, and cook for an additional 2-3 minutes.

5. Remove from heat and garnish with sesame seeds and chopped green onions if desired.

6. Serve over cooked quinoa or brown rice if desired.

Cooking Time: 15 minutes

7. Spinach and Feta Stuffed Chicken Breast

These spinach and feta stuffed chicken breasts make a flavorful and protein-packed lunch option for your IVF diet.

Ingredients:

- 2 boneless, skinless chicken breasts
- 1 cup fresh spinach leaves
- 1/2 cup crumbled feta cheese

- 2 cloves garlic, minced
- Salt and pepper to taste
- Olive oil for cooking

Instructions:

1. Preheat the oven to 375°F (190°C).

2. Butterfly the chicken breasts by slicing them horizontally but not all the way through.

3. Season the inside with salt and pepper.

4. Stuff each chicken breast with fresh spinach, crumbled feta, and minced garlic.

5. Heat olive oil in an oven-safe skillet over medium-high heat.

6. Sear the stuffed chicken breasts for about 2 minutes on each side until golden brown.

7. Transfer the skillet to the preheated oven and bake for 15-20 minutes or until the chicken is cooked through and no longer pink in the center.

8. Serve hot.

Cooking Time: 30 minutes

8. Lentil and Vegetable Curry

This hearty lentil and vegetable curry is rich in plant-based protein and flavor, perfect for an IVF diet lunch.

Ingredients:

- 1 cup dried green or brown lentils, rinsed and drained
- 2 cups vegetable broth
- 1 cup diced carrots
- 1 cup diced potatoes
- 1 cup diced bell peppers
- 1 cup diced onion
- 2 cloves garlic, minced
- 1 tablespoon olive oil
- 2 tablespoons curry powder
- Salt and pepper to taste
- Fresh cilantro leaves for garnish (optional)

Instructions:

1. In a large pot, heat olive oil over medium heat.

2. Add diced onion, carrots, potatoes, and bell peppers. Sauté until onions are translucent.

3. Stir in minced garlic and curry powder, cooking for another minute.

4. Add lentils, vegetable broth, salt, and pepper.

5. Bring to a boil, then reduce heat, cover, and simmer for about 25-30 minutes, or until lentils and vegetables are tender.

6. Garnish with fresh cilantro leaves if desired.

7. Serve with brown rice or whole-grain naan bread if desired.

Cooking Time: 40 minutes

9. Chickpea and Avocado Salad

A chickpea and avocado salad is a refreshing and protein-rich lunch option for your IVF diet.

Ingredients:

- 1 can (15 oz) chickpeas, drained and rinsed
- 2 ripe avocados, diced
- 1 cup cherry tomatoes, halved
- 1/4 cup diced red onion
- 1/4 cup chopped fresh cilantro
- Juice of 1 lime
- 2 tablespoons olive oil

-   Salt and pepper to taste

Instructions:

1. In a large bowl, combine chickpeas, diced avocados, cherry tomatoes, diced red onion, and fresh cilantro.

2. In a small bowl, whisk together lime juice, olive oil, salt, and pepper.

3. Pour the dressing over the salad and toss to combine.

4. Serve chilled.

Cooking Time: None

10. Turkey Chili

Turkey chili is a hearty and protein-packed lunch option that's perfect for your IVF diet.

Ingredients:

-   1 lb lean ground turkey
-   1 can (15 oz) kidney beans, drained and rinsed
-   1 can (15 oz) diced tomatoes
-   1 cup diced bell peppers (any color)
-   1 cup diced onion

- 2 cloves garlic, minced
- 2 tablespoons chili powder
- 1 teaspoon cumin
- 1/2 teaspoon paprika
- Salt and pepper to taste
- Olive oil for cooking
- Optional toppings: shredded cheese, chopped green onions, Greek yogurt

Instructions:

1. In a large pot, heat olive oil over medium heat.

2. Add diced onion and bell peppers and sauté until softened.

3. Add minced garlic and cook for another minute.

4. Add ground turkey and cook until browned, breaking it apart with a spoon.

5. Stir in chili powder, cumin, paprika, salt, and pepper.

6. Add diced tomatoes and kidney beans.

7. Bring to a simmer and cook for about 15-20 minutes.

8. Serve hot with optional toppings if desired.

Cooking Time: 30 minutes

CHAPTER FOUR

IVF Diet Dinner Recipes

1. Baked Salmon with Lemon and Asparagus

This baked salmon and asparagus dinner is rich in omega-3 fatty acids and vitamins, making it an excellent choice for an IVF diet.

Ingredients:

- 2 salmon fillets
- 1 bunch asparagus
- 1 lemon, sliced
- 2 cloves garlic, minced
- 2 tablespoons olive oil
- Salt and pepper to taste
- Fresh dill for garnish (optional)

Instructions:

1. Preheat the oven to 375°F (190°C).

2. Place salmon fillets on a baking sheet.

3. Arrange asparagus around the salmon.

4. Drizzle olive oil over salmon and asparagus, then sprinkle minced garlic, salt, and pepper.

5. Place lemon slices on top of the salmon.

6. Bake for about 15-20 minutes or until the salmon flakes easily with a fork and asparagus is tender.

7. Garnish with fresh dill if desired.

8. Serve hot.

Cooking Time: 20 minutes

2. Quinoa and Black Bean Stuffed Bell Peppers

These quinoa and black bean stuffed bell peppers are a protein-rich and fiber-packed dinner option for your IVF diet.

Ingredients:

- 4 large bell peppers (any color)
- 1 cup cooked quinoa
- 1 can (15 oz) black beans, drained and rinsed
- 1 cup diced tomatoes
- 1/2 cup diced red onion
- 1/2 cup corn kernels (fresh, frozen, or canned)
- 1 teaspoon chili powder
- Salt and pepper to taste

- 1 cup shredded cheese (optional)

Instructions:

1. Preheat the oven to 375°F (190°C).

2. Cut the tops off the bell peppers and remove seeds and membranes.

3. In a large bowl, combine cooked quinoa, black beans, diced tomatoes, diced red onion, corn kernels, chili powder, salt, and pepper.

4. Stuff each bell pepper with the quinoa and black bean mixture.

5. If using cheese, sprinkle it on top of each stuffed pepper.

6. Place the stuffed peppers in a baking dish and cover with foil.

7. Bake for about 25-30 minutes or until the peppers are tender.

8. Serve hot.

Cooking Time: 30 minutes

3. Grilled Chicken with Quinoa and Roasted Vegetables

This grilled chicken with quinoa and roasted vegetables is a well-rounded and nutritious dinner choice for your IVF diet.

Ingredients:

- 2 boneless, skinless chicken breasts
- 1 cup cooked quinoa
- 2 cups mixed vegetables (e.g., bell peppers, zucchini, cherry tomatoes)
- 2 tablespoons olive oil
- 1 teaspoon Italian seasoning (or your favorite seasoning blend)
- Salt and pepper to taste
- Lemon wedges for garnish (optional)

Instructions:

1. Preheat the grill to medium-high heat.

2. Season chicken breasts with olive oil, Italian seasoning, salt, and pepper.

3. Grill chicken for about 6-8 minutes per side or until

cooked through.

4. While chicken is grilling, toss mixed vegetables with olive oil, salt, and pepper.

5. Place vegetables on a grill basket or skewers and grill for about 5-7 minutes or until tender and slightly charred.

6. Serve grilled chicken on a bed of cooked quinoa, with roasted vegetables on the side.

7. Garnish with lemon wedges if desired.

8. Serve hot.

Cooking Time: 20 minutes

4. Spinach and Mushroom Stuffed Pork Tenderloin

This spinach and mushroom stuffed pork tenderloin is a flavorful and protein-packed dinner choice for your IVF diet.

Ingredients:

- 1 pork tenderloin (about 1 lb)
- 2 cups fresh spinach leaves
- 1 cup sliced mushrooms

- 2 cloves garlic, minced
- 1/4 cup shredded mozzarella cheese (optional)
- 2 tablespoons olive oil
- Salt and pepper to taste

Instructions:

1. Preheat the oven to 375°F (190°C).

2. Butterfly the pork tenderloin by slicing it horizontally but not all the way through.

3. Season the inside with salt and pepper.

4. In a skillet, heat olive oil over medium heat.

5. Sauté sliced mushrooms until they release moisture and become tender.

6. Add minced garlic and fresh spinach, cooking until wilted.

7. Lay the sautéed spinach and mushrooms on the inside of the pork tenderloin.

8. If using cheese, sprinkle it on top of the spinach and mushrooms.

9. Roll up the pork tenderloin and secure with kitchen twine.

10. Place the stuffed pork tenderloin on a baking sheet.

11. Roast for about 25-30 minutes or until the internal temperature reaches 145°F (63°C).

12. Let it rest for a few minutes before slicing.

13. Serve hot.

Cooking Time: 30 minutes

5. Baked Cod with Quinoa and Roasted Broccoli

This baked cod with quinoa and roasted broccoli is a balanced and nutritious IVF diet dinner option.

Ingredients:

- 2 cod fillets
- 1 cup cooked quinoa
- 2 cups broccoli florets
- 2 tablespoons olive oil
- Juice of 1 lemon
- 2 cloves garlic, minced
- Salt and pepper to taste

Instructions:

1. Preheat the oven to 375°F (190°C).

2. In a bowl, combine broccoli florets with olive oil, minced garlic, salt, and pepper.

3. Spread the broccoli on a baking sheet.

4. Season cod fillets with olive oil, lemon juice, salt, and pepper.

5. Place the cod fillets on the same baking sheet as the broccoli.

6. Bake for about 15-20 minutes or until the cod flakes easily with a fork and the broccoli is tender.

7. Serve cod over cooked quinoa with roasted broccoli on the side.

8. Drizzle with additional lemon juice if desired.

9. Serve hot.

Cooking Time: 20 minutes

6. Tofu Stir-Fry with Brown Rice

This tofu stir-fry with brown rice is a delicious and protein-rich dinner option suitable for your IVF diet.

Ingredients:

- 1 block (14 oz) firm tofu, cubed

- 2 cups mixed vegetables (e.g., bell peppers, broccoli, carrots)

- 1 cup cooked brown rice

- 2 tablespoons low-sodium soy sauce or tamari

- 1 tablespoon sesame oil

- 2 cloves garlic, minced

- 1 teaspoon grated ginger

- Salt and pepper to taste

Instructions:

1. In a large skillet or wok, heat sesame oil over medium-high heat.

2. Add minced garlic and grated ginger and stir-fry for about 30 seconds.

3. Add mixed vegetables and tofu cubes.

4. Stir-fry until vegetables are tender and tofu is slightly browned.

5. Stir in soy sauce, salt, and pepper.

6. Serve tofu stir-fry over cooked brown rice.

7. Garnish with chopped green onions if desired.

8. Serve hot.

Cooking Time: 20 minutes (for brown rice)

7. Beef or Plant-Based Patty with Lettuce Wrap and Sweet Potato Fries

These lettuce wrap patties with sweet potato fries offer a satisfying and low-carb dinner option for your IVF diet.

Ingredients:

- 2 beef or plant-based burger patties
- Large lettuce leaves (e.g., iceberg or romaine)

- 2 sweet potatoes, cut into fries

- 2 tablespoons olive oil

- Salt and pepper to taste

- Optional toppings: sliced tomato, onion, avocado

Instructions:

1. Preheat the oven to 425°F (220°C).

2. Toss sweet potato fries with olive oil, salt, and pepper.

3. Spread sweet potato fries on a baking sheet.

4. Bake for about 20-25 minutes or until fries are crispy, flipping halfway through.

5. While fries are baking, cook burger patties according to package instructions (grill, stovetop, or oven).

6. Place each cooked patty on a large lettuce leaf.

7. Add optional toppings if desired.

8. Serve with sweet potato fries.

9. Serve hot.

Cooking Time: 25 minutes

8. Baked Chicken Thighs with Quinoa and Steamed Broccoli

This baked chicken thigh dinner with quinoa and steamed broccoli is a balanced and protein-rich option for your IVF diet.

Ingredients:

- 4 bone-in, skinless chicken thighs
- 1 cup cooked quinoa
- 2 cups broccoli florets
- 2 tablespoons olive oil
- Juice of 1 lemon
- 2 cloves garlic, minced
- Salt and pepper to taste

Instructions:

1. Preheat the oven to 375°F (190°C).

2. Season chicken thighs with olive oil, lemon juice, minced garlic, salt, and pepper.

3. Place chicken thighs on a baking sheet.

4. Bake for about 35-40 minutes or until chicken is cooked

through and juices run clear.

5. While chicken is baking, steam broccoli florets until tender.

6. Serve chicken thighs over cooked quinoa with steamed broccoli on the side.

7. Drizzle with additional lemon juice if desired.

8. Serve hot.

Cooking Time: 40 minutes

9. Grilled Shrimp with Quinoa and Roasted Asparagus

This grilled shrimp with quinoa and roasted asparagus dinner is a flavorful and nutrient-rich choice for your IVF diet.

Ingredients:

- 1 lb large shrimp, peeled and deveined
- 1 cup cooked quinoa
- 1 bunch asparagus
- 2 tablespoons olive oil
- Juice of 1 lemon

- 2 cloves garlic, minced

- Salt and pepper to taste

Instructions:

1. Preheat the grill to medium-high heat.

2. Season shrimp with olive oil, lemon juice, minced garlic, salt, and pepper.

3. Thread shrimp onto skewers.

4. Grill shrimp for about 2-3 minutes per side or until opaque and cooked through.

5. While shrimp is grilling, arrange asparagus on a baking sheet.

6. Drizzle with olive oil, salt, and pepper, then roast in the oven for about 10-12 minutes or until tender.

7. Serve grilled shrimp over cooked quinoa with roasted asparagus on the side.

8. Drizzle with additional lemon juice if desired.

9. Serve hot.

Cooking Time: 15 minutes

10. Beef and Vegetable Kebabs with Quinoa Pilaf

These beef and vegetable kebabs with quinoa pilaf are a satisfying and protein-rich dinner option suitable for your IVF diet.

Ingredients:

- 1 lb beef sirloin, cut into cubes
- 1 bell pepper (any color), cut into chunks
- 1 red onion, cut into chunks
- 1 zucchini, sliced
- 1 cup cooked quinoa
- 2 tablespoons olive oil
- 1 teaspoon dried oregano
- Salt and pepper to taste
- Wooden skewers, soaked in water

Instructions:

1. Preheat the grill to medium-high heat.

2. Season beef cubes with olive oil, dried oregano, salt, and pepper.

3. Thread beef, bell pepper, red onion, and zucchini onto wooden skewers.

4. Grill kebabs for about 8-10 minutes, turning occasionally, until beef is cooked to your desired level of doneness.

5. While kebabs are grilling, toss cooked quinoa with olive oil, salt, and pepper.

6. Serve beef and vegetable kebabs over quinoa pilaf.

7. Serve hot.

Cooking Time: 10 minutes (for quinoa)

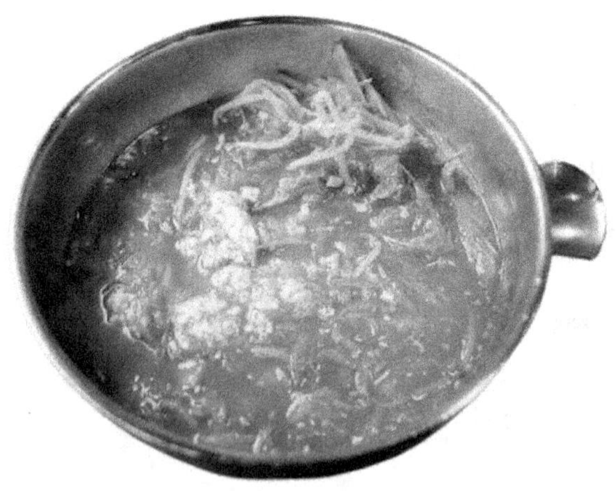

IVF Diet Snacks Recipes

1. Greek Yogurt and Berry Parfait

This Greek yogurt and berry parfait is a protein-rich and antioxidant-packed snack for your IVF diet.

Ingredients:

- 1 cup Greek yogurt
- 1/2 cup mixed berries (fresh or frozen)
- 1 tablespoon honey or maple syrup
- 1/4 cup granola

Instructions:

1. In a glass or bowl, layer Greek yogurt, mixed berries, and honey or maple syrup.

2. Top with granola for added texture and crunch.

3. Enjoy immediately.

Preparation Time: 5 minutes

2. Hummus and Veggie Sticks

Hummus and veggie sticks provide a satisfying snack rich in fiber and protein.

Ingredients:

- 1/2 cup hummus (store-bought or homemade)
- Assorted veggie sticks (carrots, cucumbers, bell peppers and celery)

Instructions:

1. Wash and cut assorted veggies into sticks.

2. Serve with hummus as a dip.

3. Enjoy as a nutritious and crunchy snack.

Preparation Time: 10 minutes (if making hummus)

3. Cottage Cheese with Pineapple

Cottage cheese with pineapple is a protein-packed and sweet snack option for your IVF diet.

Ingredients:

- 1/2 cup low-fat cottage cheese
- 1/2 cup diced fresh pineapple

Instructions:

1. In a bowl, combine cottage cheese and diced pineapple.

2. Mix well and enjoy as a creamy and satisfying snack.

Preparation Time: 5 minutes

4. Almond and Berry Trail Mix

Almond and berry trail mix is a nutrient-dense snack loaded with healthy fats, fiber, and antioxidants.

Ingredients:

- 1/4 cup almonds
- 1/4 cup dried cranberries
- 1/4 cup dried blueberries
- 1/4 cup roasted pumpkin seeds (pepitas)
- 1/4 cup dark chocolate chips (optional)

Instructions:

1. In a bowl, combine almonds, dried cranberries, dried blueberries, roasted pumpkin seeds, and dark chocolate chips if desired.

2. Mix well and portion into small snack-sized bags for convenient on-the-go snacking.

Preparation Time: 5 minutes

5. Apple Slices with Almond Butter

Apple slices with almond butter make for a satisfying and fiber-rich snack.

Ingredients:

- 1 apple, sliced
- 2 tablespoons almond butter (or your favorite nut butter)

Instructions:

1. Slice the apple into thin rounds or wedges.

2. Dip apple slices into almond butter.

3. Enjoy this crunchy and creamy snack.

Preparation Time: 5 minutes

6. Rice Cakes with Avocado and Cherry Tomatoes

Rice cakes with avocado and cherry tomatoes provide a balanced and savory snack option.

Ingredients:

- 2 rice cakes
- 1 ripe avocado, mashed
- 1/2 cup cherry tomatoes, halved
- Salt and pepper to taste

Instructions:

1. Spread mashed avocado evenly on rice cakes.

2. Top with halved cherry tomatoes.

3. Season with salt and pepper.

4. Enjoy these crispy and creamy snacks.

Preparation Time: 5 minutes

7. Edamame with Sea Salt

Edamame with sea salt is a protein-packed and satisfying snack that's easy to prepare.

Ingredients:

- 1 cup frozen edamame pods
- Sea salt for sprinkling

Instructions:

1. Steam or boil the edamame pods according to package instructions.

2. Drain and sprinkle with sea salt.

3. Enjoy these protein-rich, lightly salted snacks.

Preparation Time: 10 minutes

8. Cucumber and Tuna Bites

Cucumber and tuna bites offer a low-carb and protein-rich snack option.

Ingredients:

- 1 cucumber, sliced into rounds
- 1 can (5 oz) tuna in water, drained
- 2 tablespoons Greek yogurt or mayonnaise
- 1/4 cup diced red onion
- Salt and pepper to taste

Instructions:

1. In a bowl, combine drained tuna, Greek yogurt or mayonnaise, diced red onion, salt, and pepper.

2. Spoon the tuna mixture onto cucumber rounds.

3. Enjoy these refreshing and savory bites.

Preparation Time: 10 minutes

9. Whole-Grain Crackers with Avocado and Salsa

Whole-grain crackers with avocado and salsa make for a crunchy and flavorful snack.

Ingredients:

- 6 whole-grain crackers
- 1 ripe avocado, sliced
- 1/2 cup salsa

Instructions:

1. Place avocado slices on each cracker.

2. Top with salsa for added flavor.

3. Enjoy this balanced and satisfying snack.

Preparation Time: 5 minutes

10. Baked Sweet Potato Fries

Baked sweet potato fries are a nutritious and flavorful snack that's easy to prepare.

Ingredients:

- 2 sweet potatoes, cut into fries
- 2 tablespoons olive oil
- Salt and paprika to taste

Instructions:

1. Preheat the oven to 425°F (220°C).

2. Toss sweet potato fries with olive oil, salt, and paprika.

3. Spread fries on a baking sheet.

4. Bake for about 25-30 minutes or until fries are crispy and golden.

5. Enjoy these naturally sweet and crunchy fries.

Preparation Time: 35 minutes

CONCLUSION

The IVF diet is a specialized dietary approach designed to support individuals and couples undergoing in vitro fertilization (IVF) treatment.

This carefully crafted diet aims to optimize fertility and increase the chances of a successful pregnancy by focusing on nutrient-rich foods, balanced macronutrients, and healthy lifestyle choices.

The fundamental principles of the IVF diet revolve around providing the body with essential nutrients that are crucial for reproductive health. These nutrients include folic acid, antioxidants, omega-3 fatty acids, and a variety of vitamins and minerals.

incorporating foods rich in these nutrients, individuals can enhance their reproductive potential and create a more favorable environment for conception and embryo development.

One of the key aspects of the IVF diet is maintaining a healthy weight. Obesity or being underweight can negatively impact fertility. Therefore, the diet encourages achieving and maintaining a healthy body weight through portion control and balanced eating.

The IVF diet also emphasizes the importance of managing stress and adopting a healthy lifestyle. High-stress levels can interfere with fertility, and stress-reduction techniques such as yoga, meditation, and regular exercise are encouraged as part of the diet plan.

Furthermore, the IVF diet recognizes the role of certain foods in promoting hormonal balance and reducing inflammation. By choosing whole grains, lean proteins, fruits, and vegetables, individuals can create a foundation of health that supports their IVF journey.

In conclusion, the IVF diet is a holistic approach to fertility that combines nutritious eating, lifestyle modifications, and stress management. While it cannot guarantee a successful outcome, it can significantly improve the chances of a healthy pregnancy during IVF treatment.

Ultimately, the IVF diet empowers individuals to take an active role in their reproductive health and provides a solid foundation for a successful fertility journey.